TABLE OF CONTENTS

INTRODUCTION

Gestational diabetes mellitus (GDM) is a type of diabetes that develops during pregnancy. It is characterized by high blood sugar levels that begin or are first recognized during pregnancy. Gestational diabetes can affect the health of both the mother and the baby if not properly managed.

During pregnancy, the body undergoes hormonal changes that can affect the way insulin, a hormone that regulates blood sugar, works. In some cases, the body may not be able to produce enough insulin to meet the increased demands, leading to elevated blood sugar levels.

Here are some key points about gestational diabetes:

Screening and Diagnosis: Pregnant women are typically screened for gestational diabetes between 24 and 28 weeks of pregnancy. Screening involves a glucose challenge test, and if the results are elevated, a follow-up glucose tolerance test may be conducted to confirm the diagnosis.

Risk Factors: Certain factors increase the risk of developing gestational diabetes, including being overweight, having a family history of diabetes, being older than 25, and belonging to certain ethnic groups.

Effects on the Mother: Gestational diabetes increases the risk of complications for the mother, including high blood pressure, preeclampsia, and the need for a cesarean section.

Effects on the Baby: Untreated or poorly managed gestational diabetes can lead to complications for the baby, such as excessive birth weight, preterm birth, respiratory distress syndrome, and an increased risk of developing type 2 diabetes later in life.

Management: The primary goal of managing gestational diabetes is to control blood sugar levels to ensure a healthy pregnancy and delivery. This typically involves lifestyle changes, including a balanced diet, regular physical activity, and, in some cases, insulin therapy or oral medications.

Monitoring: Women with gestational diabetes will need to monitor their blood sugar levels regularly, usually through a combination of self-monitoring at home and periodic checks at the healthcare provider's office.

Postpartum Monitoring: After giving birth, blood sugar levels usually return to normal. However, women who have had gestational diabetes are at an increased risk of developing type 2 diabetes later in life. Therefore, postpartum monitoring and lifestyle modifications are important to reduce this risk.

It's important for pregnant individuals to work closely with their healthcare team to manage gestational diabetes effectively and ensure a healthy pregnancy and delivery. Regular prenatal care, a balanced lifestyle, and adherence to medical recommendations are crucial components of managing gestational diabetes.

SYMPTOMS GESTATIONAL DIABETES

Gestational diabetes often doesn't cause noticeable symptoms, and that's why it's crucial for pregnant individuals to undergo screening during routine prenatal care. However, in some cases, women may experience symptoms similar to those of regular diabetes. These symptoms may include:

Increased Thirst: Feeling unusually thirsty and drinking more fluids than usual.

Frequent Urination: Needing to urinate more frequently, especially during the night.

Fatigue: Feeling more tired than usual, which can be a symptom of elevated blood sugar levels.

It's important to note that these symptoms are not unique to gestational diabetes and can occur for various reasons during pregnancy. Since gestational diabetes often doesn't present with noticeable symptoms, routine screening becomes crucial for early detection and management.

During prenatal care, healthcare providers typically conduct a glucose challenge test around 24 to 28 weeks of pregnancy to screen for gestational diabetes. If the results are elevated, a follow-up glucose tolerance test may be performed to confirm the diagnosis.

If you are pregnant and experience any unusual symptoms, it's essential to discuss them with your healthcare provider. Additionally, if you have risk factors for gestational diabetes, such as being overweight or having a family history of diabetes, your healthcare provider may monitor you more closely for the condition. Early detection and management of gestational diabetes are essential for the health of both the mother and the baby.

The exact cause of gestational diabetes is not fully understood, but it is believed to be related to hormonal changes that occur during pregnancy. These changes can affect the way insulin, a hormone that regulates blood sugar, functions in the body. Here are some key factors that contribute to the development of gestational diabetes:

Hormonal Changes: During pregnancy, the placenta produces hormones that help the baby grow and develop. Some of these hormones can interfere with the action of insulin, leading to insulin resistance. Insulin resistance means that the body's cells don't respond as effectively to insulin, resulting in elevated blood sugar levels.

Increased Insulin Needs: As the pregnancy progresses, the mother's body needs more insulin to manage the increased glucose in the bloodstream and meet the needs of the growing baby. If the body is unable to produce enough insulin to compensate for this increased demand, gestational diabetes may develop.

Risk Factors: Certain factors increase the risk of developing gestational diabetes. These include being overweight or obese before pregnancy, having a family history of diabetes, being older than 25, belonging to certain ethnic groups (such as African American, Hispanic, Native American, or Asian), and having a history of gestational diabetes in a previous pregnancy.

Previous Births: Women who have previously given birth to a baby weighing 9 pounds or more or have had a stillbirth may be at an increased risk of gestational diabetes.

Polycystic Ovary Syndrome (PCOS): Women with PCOS, a condition characterized by hormonal imbalances, may have a higher risk of developing gestational diabetes.

It's important to note that gestational diabetes is a temporary condition that typically develops in the later stages of pregnancy. In most cases, blood sugar levels return to normal after childbirth. However, women who have had gestational diabetes are at an increased risk of developing type 2 diabetes later in life. Maintaining a healthy lifestyle, including regular physical activity and a balanced diet, can help reduce this risk.

Additionally, proper prenatal care, including screening and monitoring, is essential for managing gestational diabetes during pregnancy.

The treatment for gestational diabetes aims to control blood sugar levels to ensure a healthy pregnancy and reduce the risk of complications for both the mother and the baby. Treatment typically involves a combination of lifestyle changes and, in some cases, medications like insulin. Here are the key components of the treatment for gestational diabetes:

Diet and Nutrition:

Balanced Diet: Adopting a balanced diet that includes a variety of nutrient-dense foods is crucial. This may involve working with a registered dietitian to create a personalized meal plan.

Monitoring Carbohydrate Intake: Keeping track of carbohydrate intake can help manage blood sugar levels. Distributing carbohydrates evenly throughout the day and avoiding large, concentrated amounts in one meal can be beneficial.

Regular Meals and Snacks: Eating regular, smaller meals and incorporating healthy snacks can help stabilize blood sugar levels.

Physical Activity:

Regular Exercise: Engaging in regular physical activity is important for managing blood sugar levels. This could include activities like walking, swimming, or other exercises approved by the healthcare provider.

Monitoring Blood Sugar Before and After Exercise: It's important to monitor blood sugar levels before and after exercise to ensure they stay within the target range.

Blood Sugar Monitoring:

Home Monitoring: Women with gestational diabetes may be advised to monitor their blood sugar levels at home using a glucose meter. This helps track how well blood sugar levels are being managed and allows for adjustments to diet or medication if needed.

Regular Healthcare Provider Check-ups: Regular prenatal check-ups are essential for monitoring the health of both the mother and the baby. These appointments may include blood tests to assess blood sugar control.

Insulin Therapy or Medications:

Insulin Injections: In some cases, insulin therapy may be recommended to help control blood sugar levels. Insulin is safe to use during pregnancy and is usually administered through injections.

Oral Medications: While insulin is the most common medication for managing gestational diabetes, in certain situations, oral medications may be prescribed. However, not all oral medications are considered safe during pregnancy, so this decision is made on an individual basis.

Frequent Monitoring and Adjustments:

Regular Follow-up: Close monitoring and regular follow-up with healthcare providers are essential to assess the effectiveness of the treatment plan. Adjustments to the treatment plan may be made based on blood sugar monitoring results.

Postpartum Monitoring:

Monitoring After Birth: After giving birth, blood sugar levels usually return to normal. However, women who have had gestational diabetes are at an increased risk of developing type 2 diabetes. Postpartum monitoring and follow-up care are important to address any ongoing risks.

It's crucial for individuals with gestational diabetes to work closely with their healthcare team to develop and adhere to a personalized treatment plan. Effective management of gestational diabetes contributes to a healthier pregnancy and reduces the risk of complications for both the mother and the baby.

Effectively managing gestational diabetes can provide several benefits for both the mother and the baby. Here are some of the key benefits:

Reduced Risk of Complications for the Mother:

Reduced Risk of Preeclampsia: Gestational diabetes is associated with an increased risk of developing preeclampsia, a condition characterized by high blood pressure and potential organ damage. Proper management can help mitigate this risk.

Lowered Risk of Cesarean Section: Well-controlled gestational diabetes may reduce the likelihood of needing a cesarean section (C-section) delivery.

Improved Cardiovascular Health: Managing blood sugar levels during pregnancy contributes to better overall cardiovascular health for the mother.

Promotion of Healthy Fetal Development:

Normal Fetal Growth: Effective management of gestational diabetes helps regulate blood sugar levels, reducing the risk of excessive fetal growth (macrosomia). This lowers the chances of complications during delivery.

Lower Risk of Respiratory Distress Syndrome: Babies born to mothers with well-controlled gestational diabetes are less likely to experience respiratory distress syndrome, a breathing problem common in premature infants.

Prevention of Hypoglycemia in Newborns: Babies born to mothers with gestational diabetes can sometimes experience low blood sugar (hypoglycemia). Proper management helps prevent or minimize this risk.

Improved Postpartum Health:

Reduced Risk of Type 2 Diabetes: Women who effectively manage gestational diabetes are less likely to develop type 2 diabetes later in life.

Enhanced Weight Management: A focus on healthy eating and physical activity during and after pregnancy contributes to better weight management.

Positive Impact on Breastfeeding: Well-controlled gestational diabetes can positively impact breastfeeding success and the health of the newborn.

Empowerment Through Lifestyle Changes:

Healthy Habits: The lifestyle changes recommended for managing gestational diabetes, such as a balanced diet and regular exercise, promote overall health and well-being.

Educational Opportunities: Managing gestational diabetes often involves education about nutrition, blood sugar monitoring, and healthy habits. This knowledge can empower individuals to make positive choices for themselves and their families.

Enhanced Maternal and Fetal Well-being:

Reduced Stress and Anxiety: Effective management of gestational diabetes can reduce stress and anxiety associated with potential complications during pregnancy and delivery.

Optimal Health for the Baby: Well-controlled gestational diabetes supports optimal health for the baby, contributing to a positive start in life.

It's important to note that the benefits of managing gestational diabetes are closely tied to adherence to the treatment plan and regular monitoring. Women with gestational diabetes should work closely with their healthcare team to ensure the best possible outcomes for both themselves and their babies.

Here are some recipes with ingredients and basic instructions for each:

1. GRILLED LEMON HERB CHICKEN:

Ingredients:

Chicken breasts

Lemon juice

Olive oil

Garlic, minced

Fresh herbs (rosemary, thyme, or oregano)

Salt and pepper to taste

Instructions:

Combine lemon juice, olive oil, minced garlic, chopped herbs, salt, and pepper to create a marinade.

Marinate chicken breasts for at least 30 minutes.

Grill the chicken until fully cooked, approximately 6-8 minutes per side.

2. VEGETARIAN QUINOA SALAD:

Ingredients:

Quinoa

Cherry tomatoes, halved

Cucumber, diced

Red onion, finely chopped

Feta cheese, crumbled

Olive oil

Lemon juice

Fresh basil, chopped

Salt and pepper to taste

Instructions:

Cook quinoa according to package instructions and let it cool.

In a large bowl, combine quinoa, tomatoes, cucumber, red onion, and feta cheese.

In a small bowl, whisk together olive oil, lemon juice, basil, salt, and pepper. Pour over the quinoa mixture and toss.

3. SPAGHETTI BOLOGNESE:

Ingredients:

Ground beef

Onion, diced

Garlic, minced

Tomato sauce

Crushed tomatoes

Italian seasoning

Salt and pepper to taste

Spaghetti pasta

Instructions:

In a pan, brown the ground beef with diced onions and minced garlic.

Add tomato sauce, crushed tomatoes, Italian seasoning, salt, and pepper. Simmer for 20-30 minutes.

Cook spaghetti according to package instructions and serve with the Bolognese sauce.

4. MANGO AVOCADO SALSA:

Ingredients:

Mango, diced

Avocado, diced

Red onion, finely chopped

Jalapeño, minced

Fresh cilantro, chopped

Lime juice

Salt to taste

Instructions:

In a bowl, combine diced mango, avocado, red onion, jalapeño, and cilantro.

Add lime juice and salt to taste. Mix gently and refrigerate for 30 minutes before serving.

5. BAKED SALMON WITH LEMON DILL SAUCE:

Ingredients:

Salmon fillets

Lemon slices

Fresh dill, chopped

Garlic powder

Olive oil

Salt and pepper to taste

Instructions:

Preheat the oven to 375°F (190°C).

Place salmon fillets on a baking sheet. Drizzle with olive oil and sprinkle with garlic powder, salt, and pepper.

Top with lemon slices and fresh dill. Bake for 15-20 minutes or until the salmon is cooked through.

6. VEGETARIAN CHICKPEA CURRY:

Ingredients:

Chickpeas (canned or cooked)

Onion, finely chopped

Garlic, minced

Ginger, grated

Tomatoes, diced

Coconut milk

Curry powder

Cumin

Turmeric

Salt and pepper to taste

Instructions:

In a pan, sauté chopped onion, minced garlic, and grated ginger until fragrant.

Add diced tomatoes, chickpeas, coconut milk, curry powder, cumin, turmeric, salt, and pepper. Simmer for 15-20 minutes.

7. CAPRESE SALAD WITH BALSAMIC GLAZE:

Ingredients:

Fresh tomatoes, sliced

Fresh mozzarella, sliced

Fresh basil leaves

Balsamic glaze

Olive oil

Salt and pepper to taste

Instructions:

Arrange tomato and mozzarella slices on a plate.

Tuck fresh basil leaves between the slices.

Drizzle with balsamic glaze and olive oil. Season with salt and pepper.

8. STIR-FRIED TOFU AND VEGETABLES:

Ingredients:

Firm tofu, cubed

Broccoli florets

Bell peppers, sliced

Carrots, julienned

Soy sauce

Sesame oil

Garlic, minced

Ginger, grated

Green onions, chopped

Instructions:

In a wok or pan, stir-fry tofu until golden brown. Set aside.

Stir-fry broccoli, bell peppers, and carrots until crisp-tender.

Add minced garlic and grated ginger. Stir in the cooked tofu.

Drizzle with soy sauce and sesame oil. Garnish with chopped green onions.

9. LEMON GARLIC SHRIMP PASTA:

Ingredients:

Shrimp, peeled and deveined

Linguine pasta

Lemon juice

Garlic, minced

Cherry tomatoes, halved

Fresh parsley, chopped

Olive oil

Salt and pepper to taste

Instructions:

Cook linguine according to package instructions.

In a pan, sauté shrimp in olive oil and minced garlic until pink.

Add lemon juice, cherry tomatoes, salt, and pepper. Toss with cooked pasta. Garnish with fresh parsley.

10. CAULIFLOWER AND CHICKPEA CURRY:

Ingredients:

Cauliflower, cut into florets

Chickpeas (canned or cooked)

Onion, finely chopped

Tomato puree

Coconut milk

Curry powder

Cumin

Coriander

Turmeric

Garlic, minced

Ginger, grated

Salt and pepper to taste

Instructions:

Sauté chopped onion, minced garlic, and grated ginger in a pot until softened.

Add cauliflower florets, chickpeas, tomato puree, coconut milk, curry powder, cumin, coriander, turmeric, salt, and pepper. Simmer until cauliflower is tender.

11. MUSHROOM AND SPINACH STUFFED CHICKEN BREAST:

Ingredients:

Chicken breasts

Mushrooms, finely chopped

Spinach, chopped

Garlic, minced

Feta cheese, crumbled

Olive oil

Salt and pepper to taste

Instructions:

Preheat the oven to 375°F (190°C).

In a pan, sauté mushrooms, spinach, and garlic in olive oil until softened. Let it cool.

Cut a pocket into each chicken breast and stuff with the mushroom and spinach mixture.

Season the chicken with salt and pepper. Bake for 25-30 minutes or until cooked through.

12. BLACK BEAN AND CORN SALSA:

Ingredients:

Black beans (canned), drained and rinsed

Corn kernels (fresh or frozen), cooked

Red onion, finely chopped

Jalapeño, minced

Fresh cilantro, chopped

Lime juice

Cumin

Salt and pepper to taste

Instructions:

In a bowl, combine black beans, corn, red onion, jalapeño, and cilantro.

Add lime juice, cumin, salt, and pepper. Mix well and refrigerate before serving.

13. SHEET PAN BAKED PARMESAN CRUSTED SALMON AND VEGETABLES:

Ingredients:

Salmon fillets

Asparagus, trimmed

Cherry tomatoes, halved

Parmesan cheese, grated

Lemon juice

Olive oil

Garlic powder

Salt and pepper to taste

Instructions:

Preheat the oven to 400°F (200°C).

Place salmon, asparagus, and cherry tomatoes on a baking sheet.

Drizzle with olive oil and lemon juice. Sprinkle Parmesan, garlic powder, salt, and pepper.

Bake for 15-20 minutes or until the salmon is cooked and the vegetables are tender.

14. PESTO PASTA WITH CHERRY TOMATOES AND MOZZARELLA:

Ingredients:

Pasta (penne or your choice)

Cherry tomatoes, halved

Fresh mozzarella, diced

Pesto sauce

Olive oil

Basil leaves, for garnish

Salt and pepper to taste

Instructions:

Cook pasta according to package instructions. Drain and set aside.

In a bowl, combine pasta, cherry tomatoes, mozzarella, and pesto sauce.

Drizzle with olive oil, season with salt and pepper, and garnish with fresh basil leaves.

15. TERIYAKI CHICKEN STIR-FRY:

Ingredients:

Chicken breast, thinly sliced

Broccoli florets

Bell peppers, sliced

Carrots, julienned

Teriyaki sauce

Soy sauce

Garlic, minced

Ginger, grated

Sesame oil

Green onions, chopped

Instructions:

In a wok or pan, stir-fry sliced chicken until cooked through.

Add broccoli, bell peppers, and julienned carrots. Stir-fry until vegetables are crisp-tender.

In a small bowl, mix teriyaki sauce, soy sauce, minced garlic, grated ginger, and sesame oil. Pour over the chicken and vegetables. Stir until well coated.

Garnish with chopped green onions before serving.

16. EGG FRIED RICE:

Ingredients:

Cooked white rice, cooled

Eggs, beaten

Carrots, finely diced

Peas

Green onions, chopped

Soy sauce

Sesame oil

Garlic powder

Salt and pepper to taste

Instructions:

In a large pan or wok, scramble eggs in sesame oil.

Add carrots, peas, and green onions. Stir-fry until vegetables are tender.

Add cooked rice, soy sauce, garlic powder, salt, and pepper. Mix well and cook until heated through.

17. CRISPY BAKED ZUCCHINI FRIES:

Ingredients:

Zucchini, cut into fries

Panko breadcrumbs

Parmesan cheese, grated

Egg

Garlic powder

Paprika

Salt and pepper to taste

Instructions:

Preheat the oven to 425°F (220°C).

Dip zucchini fries in beaten egg and coat with a mixture of Panko breadcrumbs, Parmesan, garlic powder, paprika, salt, and pepper.

Place on a baking sheet and bake for 20-25 minutes or until golden and crispy.

18. MEDITERRANEAN QUINOA SALAD:

Ingredients:

Quinoa, cooked

Cherry tomatoes, halved

Cucumber, diced

Kalamata olives, sliced

Red onion, finely chopped

Feta cheese, crumbled

Olive oil

Lemon juice

Fresh oregano, chopped

Salt and pepper to taste

Instructions:

In a large bowl, combine cooked quinoa, tomatoes, cucumber, olives, red onion, and feta cheese.

In a small bowl, whisk together olive oil, lemon juice, oregano, salt, and pepper. Pour over the quinoa mixture and toss.

19. HONEY GARLIC GLAZED SALMON:

Ingredients:

Salmon fillets

Honey

Soy sauce

Garlic, minced

Ginger, grated

Sesame seeds

Green onions, chopped

Salt and pepper to taste

Instructions:

In a bowl, mix honey, soy sauce, minced garlic, grated ginger, sesame seeds, salt, and pepper.

Place salmon fillets in a baking dish and pour the honey garlic mixture over them.

Bake at 375°F (190°C) for 15-20 minutes or until salmon is cooked through. Garnish with chopped green onions.

20. CAULIFLOWER PIZZA CRUST:

Ingredients:

Cauliflower, grated

Mozzarella cheese, shredded

Egg

Italian seasoning

Tomato sauce

Your favorite pizza toppings

Instructions:

Preheat the oven to 425°F (220°C).

Mix grated cauliflower with shredded mozzarella, beaten egg, and Italian seasoning.

Press the mixture onto a baking sheet to form a crust. Bake for 15-20 minutes.

Remove from the oven, add tomato sauce and your favorite toppings, then bake for an additional 10-15 minutes.

21. VEGETARIAN LENTIL SOUP:

Ingredients:

Green or brown lentils, rinsed

Onion, diced

Carrots, diced

Celery, diced

Garlic, minced

Vegetable broth

Canned diced tomatoes

Cumin

Coriander

Paprika

Bay leaves

Salt and pepper to taste

Fresh parsley, chopped (for garnish)

Instructions:

In a large pot, sauté onions, carrots, celery, and garlic until softened.

Add lentils, vegetable broth, diced tomatoes, cumin, coriander, paprika, bay leaves, salt, and pepper. Simmer for 25-30 minutes.

Garnish with fresh parsley before serving.

22. SHRIMP AND AVOCADO SALAD:

Ingredients:

Shrimp, cooked and peeled

Avocado, diced

Cherry tomatoes, halved

Red onion, finely chopped

Cilantro, chopped

Lime juice

Olive oil

Salt and pepper to taste

Instructions:

In a bowl, combine shrimp, diced avocado, cherry tomatoes, red onion, and cilantro.

Drizzle with lime juice and olive oil. Season with salt and pepper. Toss gently and serve.

23. PESTO CHICKEN PENNE PASTA:

Ingredients:

Chicken breast, sliced

Penne pasta

Cherry tomatoes, halved

Pesto sauce

Parmesan cheese, grated

Olive oil

Garlic, minced

Salt and pepper to taste

Instructions:

Cook penne pasta according to package instructions.

In a pan, sauté sliced chicken in olive oil and minced garlic until cooked.

Combine cooked pasta, chicken, cherry tomatoes, pesto sauce, and Parmesan cheese. Season with salt and pepper.

24. BAKED SWEET POTATO FRIES:

Ingredients:

Sweet potatoes, cut into fries

Olive oil

Paprika

Garlic powder

Salt and pepper to taste

Instructions:

Preheat the oven to 425°F (220°C).

Toss sweet potato fries in olive oil, paprika, garlic powder, salt, and pepper.

Spread on a baking sheet and bake for 25-30 minutes or until golden and crispy.

25. MANGO COCONUT CHIA PUDDING:

Ingredients:

Chia seeds

Coconut milk

Mango, diced

Honey or maple syrup (optional)

Shredded coconut (for garnish)

Instructions:

In a jar or bowl, mix chia seeds with coconut milk. Let it sit in the refrigerator for at least 4 hours or overnight.

Layer the chia pudding with diced mango. Optionally, drizzle with honey or maple syrup and garnish with shredded coconut.

26. LEMON GARLIC BUTTER SHRIMP:

Ingredients:

Shrimp, peeled and deveined

Butter

Garlic, minced

Lemon juice

Fresh parsley, chopped

Salt and pepper to taste

Instructions:

In a pan, melt butter and sauté minced garlic until fragrant.

Add shrimp, cook until pink and opaque.

Drizzle with lemon juice, sprinkle with chopped parsley, and season with salt and pepper.

27. VEGETABLE AND TOFU STIR-FRY:

Ingredients:

Firm tofu, cubed

Broccoli florets

Snap peas

Bell peppers, sliced

Carrots, julienned

Soy sauce

Sesame oil

Ginger, grated

Garlic, minced

Green onions, chopped

Instructions:

In a wok, stir-fry tofu until golden. Set aside.

Stir-fry broccoli, snap peas, bell peppers, and carrots until crisp-tender.

Add tofu back to the wok, drizzle with soy sauce, sesame oil, grated ginger, and minced garlic. Garnish with chopped green onions.

28. CAPRESE STUFFED PORTOBELLO MUSHROOMS:

Ingredients:

Portobello mushrooms

Tomato, sliced

Fresh mozzarella, sliced

Fresh basil leaves

Balsamic glaze

Olive oil

Salt and pepper to taste

Instructions:

Clean and remove stems from Portobello mushrooms.

Fill each mushroom with sliced tomatoes, mozzarella, and fresh basil leaves.

Drizzle with balsamic glaze and olive oil. Season with salt and pepper. Bake until cheese is melted.

29. TERIYAKI VEGGIE AND CHICKEN SKEWERS:

Ingredients:

Chicken breast, cubed

Bell peppers, assorted colors, sliced

Red onion, sliced

Zucchini, sliced

Teriyaki sauce

Olive oil

Garlic powder

Salt and pepper to taste

Instructions:

Thread chicken and vegetables onto skewers.

Mix teriyaki sauce with olive oil, garlic powder, salt, and pepper.

Brush skewers with the teriyaki mixture and grill or bake until chicken is cooked through.

30. GREEK YOGURT PARFAIT WITH BERRIES AND GRANOLA:

Ingredients:

Greek yogurt

Mixed berries (strawberries, blueberries, raspberries)

Granola

Honey

Mint leaves (optional)

Instructions:

In a glass or bowl, layer Greek yogurt with mixed berries and granola.

Drizzle with honey and garnish with mint leaves if desired.

31. CRISPY BAKED CHICKEN WINGS:

Ingredients:

Chicken wings

Baking powder

Salt and pepper to taste

Your favorite wing sauce (e.g., buffalo, barbecue)

Instructions:

Preheat the oven to 425°F (220°C).

Pat dry chicken wings and toss in a mixture of baking powder, salt, and pepper.

Place wings on a baking sheet and bake until crispy.

Toss wings in your favorite sauce before serving.

32. VEGETARIAN BUTTERNUT SQUASH AND SAGE RISOTTO:

Ingredients:

Arborio rice

Butternut squash, diced

Vegetable broth

White wine

Onion, finely chopped

Fresh sage leaves

Parmesan cheese, grated

Butter

Salt and pepper to taste

Instructions:

Sauté chopped onion in butter until translucent.

Add Arborio rice and cook until lightly toasted.

Stir in diced butternut squash, fresh sage leaves, and white wine.

Gradually add vegetable broth, stirring continuously, until the rice is creamy and cooked. Stir in Parmesan cheese, salt, and pepper.

33. MEDITERRANEAN CHICKPEA SALAD:

Ingredients:

Chickpeas (canned), drained

Cucumber, diced

Cherry tomatoes, halved

Red onion, finely chopped

Kalamata olives, sliced

Feta cheese, crumbled

Olive oil

Lemon juice

Oregano

Salt and pepper to taste

Instructions:

In a bowl, combine chickpeas, cucumber, cherry tomatoes, red onion, olives, and feta cheese.

Drizzle with olive oil and lemon juice. Sprinkle with oregano, salt, and pepper. Toss gently.

34. CAJUN SHRIMP AND SAUSAGE SKILLET:

Ingredients:

Shrimp, peeled and deveined

Smoked sausage, sliced

Bell peppers, sliced

Onion, sliced

Cajun seasoning

Garlic powder

Paprika

Olive oil

Salt and pepper to taste

Instructions:

In a skillet, sauté sliced sausage in olive oil until browned.

Add shrimp, bell peppers, and onion. Season with Cajun seasoning, garlic powder, paprika, salt, and pepper.

Cook until shrimp is pink and vegetables are tender.

35. CHOCOLATE AVOCADO MOUSSE:

Ingredients:

Ripe avocados

Cocoa powder

Maple syrup or honey

Vanilla extract

Almond milk (or any milk of choice)

Instructions:

Blend ripe avocados, cocoa powder, maple syrup or honey, and vanilla extract until smooth.

Gradually add almond milk until you achieve a creamy consistency.

Refrigerate for at least 1 hour before serving. Garnish with berries or nuts if desired.

36. STUFFED BELL PEPPERS:

Ingredients:

Bell peppers

Ground beef or turkey

Cooked rice

Onion, finely chopped

Garlic, minced

Tomato sauce

Italian seasoning

Salt and pepper to taste

Shredded cheese (optional)

Instructions:

Cut bell peppers in half and remove seeds.

In a pan, brown ground meat with onion and garlic.

Mix in cooked rice, tomato sauce, Italian seasoning, salt, and pepper.

Stuff bell peppers with the mixture and bake until peppers are tender. Optionally, top with shredded cheese before serving.

37. SHRIMP AND BROCCOLI STIR-FRY:

Ingredients:

Shrimp, peeled and deveined

Broccoli florets

Soy sauce

Ginger, grated

Garlic, minced

Sesame oil

Red pepper flakes (optional)

Rice or noodles

Instructions:

In a wok or skillet, stir-fry shrimp and broccoli in sesame oil.

Add soy sauce, grated ginger, minced garlic, and red pepper flakes.

Serve over rice or noodles.

38. QUINOA AND BLACK BEAN BURRITO BOWLS:

Ingredients:

Quinoa, cooked

Black beans (canned), drained and rinsed

Corn, cooked

Avocado, sliced

Cherry tomatoes, halved

Lime juice

Cilantro, chopped

Cumin

Salt and pepper to taste

Instructions:

Assemble bowls with quinoa, black beans, corn, avocado, and cherry tomatoes.

Drizzle with lime juice and sprinkle with chopped cilantro. Season with cumin, salt, and pepper.

39. ROASTED VEGETABLE PIZZA:

Ingredients:

Pizza dough

Tomato sauce

Mozzarella cheese, shredded

Zucchini, sliced

Bell peppers, sliced

Red onion, sliced

Cherry tomatoes, halved

Olive oil

Italian seasoning

Salt and pepper to taste

Instructions:

Roll out pizza dough and spread tomato sauce over it.

Top with shredded mozzarella, zucchini, bell peppers, red onion, and cherry tomatoes.

Drizzle with olive oil, sprinkle with Italian seasoning, salt, and pepper. Bake according to dough instructions.

40. BLUEBERRY OATMEAL MUFFINS:

Ingredients:

Rolled oats

Flour

Baking powder

Cinnamon

Eggs

Milk

Blueberries

Maple syrup or honey

Vanilla extract

Instructions:

In a bowl, mix rolled oats, flour, baking powder, and cinnamon.

In another bowl, whisk eggs, add milk, blueberries, maple syrup or honey, and vanilla extract.

Combine wet and dry ingredients, and spoon into muffin cups. Bake until a toothpick comes out clean.

NOTE: Enjoy these additional recipes! If you have any specific preferences or dietary requirements, feel free to let me know for more personalized recommendations.

CONCLUSION

In conclusion, these diverse recipes provide a wide range of options for delicious and nutritious meals across various cuisines. From flavorful and healthy salads to comforting and satisfying main dishes, these recipes offer something for everyone. Whether you're in the mood for a light and refreshing salad, a hearty stir-fry, or a sweet treat, these recipes can cater to different tastes and preferences.

Experimenting with these recipes not only introduces variety into your meals but also allows for creativity in the kitchen. Many of these dishes incorporate fresh ingredients, lean proteins, and whole grains, aligning with a balanced and wholesome approach to cooking. Additionally, the use of herbs and spices adds depth and richness to the flavors without relying heavily on excessive salt or unhealthy additives.

Remember that cooking at home provides not only the opportunity to savor delicious flavors but also the ability to control the quality of ingredients, making it a healthier and more mindful choice. Feel free to modify these recipes to suit your dietary preferences and explore the joy of creating meals that nourish both body and soul.

If you have specific dietary restrictions or preferences, or if there's a particular type of cuisine you're interested in, don't hesitate to adapt these recipes or let me know for more tailored recommendations. Happy cooking and enjoying these culinary adventures!